I0101863

Choosing meal portions

- Weight Management Series

Volume 3

Excerpt from Adopting a healthy lifestyle (1-884711-34-0)

Choosing meal portions
- Weight Management Series

- C.T. Pam

Copyright © 2013 by C. T. Pam

Published and printed in the United States by Innovative Publishers, Inc., Boston, Massachusetts.

Library of Congress Control Number: 2012922834
1-884711-64-2 978-1-884711-64-0 Paperback
Also available in the following formats
1-884711-65-0 978-1-884711-65-7 Kindle
1-884711-66-9 978-1-884711-66-4 Hardback
1-884711-67-7 978-1-884711-67-1 AudioBook
1-884711-68-5 978-1-884711-68-8 iBook
1-884711-69-3 978-1-884711-69-5 Nook

Printed in the United States of America

10 9 8 7 6 5 4 3 2 1   13 14 15 16

First edition, February 2013

For general information on our other products and services or for technical support, please contact our technical support within the United States at pub@innovative-publishers.com online at http://innovative-publishers.com.

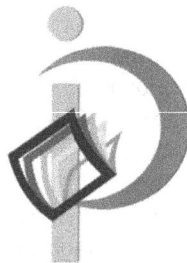

Innovative Publishers

Table of contents

Introduction to Weight Management

With the rapid rate at which obesity has spread over the last couple of decades, the importance of weight management programs has also grown as a consequence. Weight management program refers to all those activities that help an individual to either gain weight, lose weight or even to maintain it at the current level. In any of these goals, a weight management program targets increasing or maintaining the amount of lean muscle mass while decreasing the body fat percentage. Any other way of losing or gaining weight will be unhealthy in one aspect or another and may compromise health in the short term, but definitely in the long run.

Body Composition

Our body comprises of different components, namely fat, lean muscle, water, bones, organs etc. Each of them contributes to the total body weight. For each and every individual each of these constituent elements is present in different proportions. The ratio in which this distribution is present in any individual is called body composition. In the context of weight management, the division is done into two categories – fat mass and fat free mass. A healthy body composition is one in which the fat mass is low and fat free mass is higher. Through different weight management programs it is attempted to alter body composition in a manner that it boosts good health.

There are many techniques and methods to determine body composition. With technological advancements newer and more accurate equipments are available for performing body composition analysis. Traditional techniques such as skin fold measurements are easy to implement but have limited accuracy. Newer technologies such as ultrasound and bioelectric impedance analysis help in doing body composition analysis using simple and portable machines that give extremely accurate results as well. These different methods determine not only the amount of fat and lean muscle tissue but also provide a segmental analysis so that appropriate intervention strategies can be planned as part of the weight management program.

Doing body composition analysis on a regular basis should be included as part of any weight management strategy since it will help in monitoring the alterations taking place in the body as a result of the program. Since the body is undergoing change on a regular basis it is imperative that the program should also change accordingly. A program that was designed for the individual who weighed say 240 pounds will need to be changed when the person loses weight and weighs 200 pounds now. Body composition analysis also provides information on whether the weight loss is happening in a healthy manner or not. In case the weight loss happens at the expense of lean muscle or water then changes need to be done in the program so that these components can be restored to normal levels and fat loss targeted by introducing appropriate changes. A number of new age weight loss methods as well as gadgets are able to provide good results in terms of weight loss but they do it at the expense of good health. Doing a simple body composition analysis will reveal the true nature of these unhealthy methods and systems. Most new technologies also provide information on metabolic rate which is directly correlated the amount of lean mass in the body. Greater the lean mass higher will be the energy that is required by the body to maintain it. The measurement of metabolic rate helps in designing the exercise program as well as the calorie intake required as part of the diet & nutrition plan. Since the needs and requirement of each and every individual are different, the weight management strategy has to be necessarily different as well. Body composition analysis is the first step in designing a weight management program and should thereafter be done on a regular basis.

Problems with adverse body composition

A body composition analysis that reveals high fat percentage in comparison to lean muscle mass percentage points to obesity. Obesity is a modern day lifestyle disease that is essentially a silent killer. It indirectly leads to other physical as well as mental disorders, ailments and diseases that later on deplete the quality of life of the individual and in certain cases may even lead to death. The most common ailments that accompany obesity include type-2 diabetes, hypertension, cardiovascular & coronary artery disease, metabolic syndrome polycystic ovary syndrome and Dyslipidemia. Obesity also leads to gastrointestinal issues such as Cholelithiasis, GERD or Gastroesophageal Reflex Disease, Fatty Liver Disease, Colon Cancer and Hernia; genitourinary problems include erectile dysfunction, renal failure, incontinence and hypogonadism; Respiratory problems include sleep apnea, Hypoventilation syndrome and dyspnea. Apart from these physical ailments obesity also leads to psychological problems that arise from a diminished self confidence and if left unchecked may even lead to chronic depression.

Causes of Obesity

Obesity is caused by an energy intake in the form of diet that is not balanced by equivalent amount of physical activity. The basic law of conservation of energy cannot be violated at any cost and hence, energy excess will lead to weight gain while energy deficit will lead to weight loss. Energy input into the body is through the food that we eat. Energy output is the sum of a number of parameters that include – energy expended through physical exercise, energy spent in activities performed in daily life, basal metabolic rate or the energy required by the body to perform essential body functions such as respiration and digestion; in addition there are a few other parameters such as *thermic effect of food* and *adaptive thermogenesis* that add onto energy output but only in relatively small amounts. It is when the energy input becomes greater than energy output that the body starts storing this excess energy in the form of body fat. Some amount of fat is essential for efficient body functioning but when the fat percentage goes above certain levels it leads to obesity and consequently a host of other disorders and diseases.

This energy imbalance is the objective reason behind obesity but it is important to understand the underlying reasons why this imbalance is created. Imbalanced diet and sedentary lifestyle are the primary causes which get accentuated as a result of numerous personal, social, cultural and familial issues. Genetics and medical conditions also contribute towards increasing the fat mass in an individual. While most parameters seem to be alterable, some of these parameters may not seem to be in control of the individual and a situation of helplessness may be experienced. However, there are

3

ways and means to counter any of these issues that gradually lead to weight loss in a healthy manner.

Genetic factors and Body Type

As mentioned above certain parameters that influence body composition cannot be modified. Genetic predisposition is one such parameter. Genetics define the body type of an individual which then affects the way in which the body reacts to a certain lifestyle and also to any alteration that is forced on this lifestyle. There are different classification techniques for differentiating between different body types.

1. The ancient Indian science of *Ayurveda* uses a classification method based on energy patterns or types. It is believed as per *Ayurveda* that the universe comprises of five basic elements – space, air, water, fire and earth. A combination of these basic elements is responsible for defining the human physiology. The basis of classification therefore is on the basis of energy patterns or *doshas* which comprise of one or more of these elements. The three *doshas* – *vata, pitta* and *kapha* define the person's physiology and all *Ayurvedic* treatments start from the identification of the *dosha* and identifying the imbalance in the *dosha* pattern. Once this is done remedial solution can be prescribed the aim of which is to restore the balance in the elements.

2. The second classification technique is based on the metabolic type. Under this classification technique the basis of differentiation between body types is the dominating gland in the endocrine system. It is believed that the biochemical reactions happening in the body of the individual are influenced and controlled by the dominating gland. This dominance of one particular gland over the others is built into the genetic structure and has a significant impact on the metabolic processes in the body. These metabolic processes take up raw materials such as carbohydrates, fats, proteins in different proportions and occur in the presence of catalysts that are available through micronutrients such as minerals and vitamins. The difference in proportions of raw material

utilized is due to the functioning differences between these glands of the endocrine system. The classification is done into 4 main categories – adrenal (controls reaction to environmental stresses and dangers), gonad (controls reproduction and growth), thyroid (controls metabolism) and pituitary (control the secretion of all glands) depending upon the dominating gland. Different diets and exercise routines are recommended for different body types.

3. The third classification technique and most commonly used in the context of weight management programs is on the basis of Somatotype. The system is based on identifying the association between psychological behavior patterns or temperament with the body structure of the individual. Under this system it is believed that the characteristic behavioral patterns as exhibited by an individual are typical of his or her own body type to a significantly large extent. The body type as in other classification systems is genetically predetermined. People having a similar body type are expected to show similar behavioral traits under this system. The system of classification is on the basis of the 3 elements or Somatotypes that are named after cell groups known as *germinal epithelium* formed during the growth of the embryo in the womb. The three Somatotypes are named after the three germ layers - *mesoderm, endoderm* and *ectoderm* and are therefore called Mesomorph, Endomorph and Ectomorph respectively. Mesomorphs are characterized by a predominance of lean muscle, connective tissues and bone; Endomorphs are characterized by a predominant roundness & softness in the different parts of the body as a consequence of excess body fat; Ectomorphs are characterized by fragility & linearity and are therefore possess frail and weak body structures which are devoid of fat as well as lean muscle. An individual may not necessarily be a pure Somatotype and can be a combination of one or more of these Somatotypes.

These body types are not inflexible to change arising from application of stimulus in the form of exercise and diet. Not each and every one possesses a dream body shape and structure by birth. Similarly, not everyone who has the nature predisposition to a good physique is able to maintain it. The genetic code embedded into our body in the form of body type plays a significant role in determining our body shape but it is not the only parameter. It is true that an Ectomorph may ingest large number of calories as part of diet and may perform rigorous strength training routines but still may find it difficult to add an extra pound of weight. Similarly, an endomorph may perform long duration cardiovascular workouts but still may not be able to shed those extra pounds of fat stored in the body. However, genetic predisposition only indicates the difficulty to create changes; nowhere does it mention that it is impossible. Moreover, in most cases an individual is a combination of Somatotypes which makes it possible to create changes in one direction or the other depending upon the requirement. It is therefore of utmost importance to identify the body type and the goals before designing an exercise program and diet plan. Once this identification has been done, adherence to a scientifically designed weight management program will lead to achievement of the desired targets that have been set.

Components of weight management program

A healthy weight management program should be based on the four pillars of wellness – physical fitness, balanced diet & nutrition, rest & relaxation and mental attitude. A balance between all the four components is crucial for the success of a weight management program. A good fitness routine which is not accompanied by an appropriate diet will not help the individual trying to lose weight. Similarly, a person who does not have the right mental frame of mind will find it extremely difficult to adhere to certain basic restrictions that such a program may impose; as a result of which the whole program fails. A weight management program needs to be customized according the needs and goals of the individual. This customization needs to be reflected in all the components as well. In case even one of them is not in sync it can derail the whole program itself.

Balanced diet & nutrition

A good balanced and nutritious diet is paramount to the success of a weight management program. Not only should it provide the right amount of energy depending upon the goals of the program, it should also provide the necessary micronutrients in adequate quantities for long term sustainable weight loss and overall health. A balanced diet incorporates energy compounds such as carbohydrates, fats and proteins, micronutrients such as vitamins and minerals as well as fiber and water in adequate quantities. As mentioned before the quantity and proportion of the main energy compounds depends on the goal of the program while micronutrients should be available to the body as per standard guidelines such as DV (Daily Value), RDA (Recommended Dietary Allowance) and EAR (Estimated Average Requirement).

In case the goal is to lose weight then an energy deficit needs to be created in a way that energy intake is less than energy output. This may involve reducing the quantities of the energy compounds from the normal diet and vice versa in case weight gain is the goal. As part of a weight management diet plan identifying the calorie content of meals is extremely crucial. To lose one pound of fat, a deficit of 3,500 calories needs to be created. This can be done by ensuring a regular deficit of 500 calories per day throughout the week. A gradual weight loss rate of one to two pounds per week is ideal for the body since it gets time to adapt to the changed conditions. Moreover, gradual weight loss ensures that there is least amount of muscle loss that happens as part of the weight loss process. This is where the efficacy of crash diets or very low calorie diets is questioned. Apart from loss of muscle tissue they cause micronutrient deficiency extremely dangerous to overall health. Certain research studies also confirm that such diets in fact may lead to fat gain since the body experiences starvation and tends to preserve the energy dense compounds for later utilization. This is done at the expense of lean muscle tissue which is difficult to maintain in the body.

In general any meal should include around 55 to 60% energy being provided through carbohydrates, 25 to 30% energy through fats and approximately 10 to 20% through proteins. This principally ensures that while all the energy requirements are met, nourishment of the body is not compromised upon. Even in case an energy deficit is required for losing weight it created in such a way that all nutrients including fats are available to the body for essential functions that need to be performed for healthy a mind & body.

Once the energy requirements have been calculated the next step in the preparation of a balanced diet plan is identification of the meals and meal content. By identification of the meals, it is intended to finalize the meal frequency and the meal timings such that they can be incorporated in the lifestyle in an easy manner. Too many alteration in the existing pattern of life make the adherence to the plan that much more difficult. Therefore, a diet plan should be designed taking into consideration the individual's lifestyle and preferences. In this context the question of meal frequency becomes a pertinent one. The three meal plan has been ingrained into modern day diets since it is conveniently adopted into work life pattern. It may not necessarily be as good and efficient for overall health as well as for weight loss in comparison to a high frequency diet plan such as a 6 meal plan.

Our body requires energy at a particular rate; this rate is defined by our metabolic rate but there may be spikes in demand such as the post exercise period. Clearly, the body does not require energy at the rate at which we eat and the rate at which the energy is released in our body upon digestion of food. In such a situation the excess energy needs to be stored in the body to be utilized at a later stage. The body can do it in the form of glycogen in the liver and muscles but once these limited space stores are filled up then it converts the extra energy into fat which can be stored all over the body. Secondly, whenever a heavy meal is consumed the insulin spike that occurs upon increase in glucose level in the blood, stays on for a longer period of time. In a similar manner this also results in storage of carbohydrates initially as glycogen but later on as fat. Smaller meals ensure that the body gets energy at a rate commensurate to its requirements so that it does not have to convert and store it as body fat. A high frequency 6 meal plan aids in this process of immediate utilization.

The other factor is the proportion of energy that is derived from stored energy reserves versus that derived from food that has been consume in the recent past. The body stores energy compounds like glucose in the blood, glycogen or long chain glucose molecules in the liver and muscles. And fat in the adipose tissue. Whenever the requirement for energy arises the body meets it through one of these sources. When extra carbohydrates are ingested as part of the meal the body stops utilizing the fat stored in the body, on top of this, the extra carbohydrate gets converted into fat. In a high frequency meal plan, the amount of carbohydrates consumed in any meal is limited, which prevents prolonged insulin spike from occurring. This helps in preventing conversion of carbohydrates into fat and also helps in utilizing stored fat for meeting energy requirement.

As part of weight management programs high frequency smaller meals are often suggested due to the aforementioned reasons. The other psychological advantages offered by these plans are beneficial in ensuring adherence during the initial difficult periods of change. By trimming down meal quantities and increasing frequency, cravings that lead to unplanned eating can be prevented. Since, as part of the meal itself there are many meals, the meal content is pre-planned and hence, the chances of eating something unhealthy out of the diet plan are reduce. Uncontrolled hunger pangs are also not experienced since the gap between meals is shorter. This has a dual advantage – apart from preventing binge eating it also helps in avoiding overeating during the main meals. The effect of frequent meals on metabolism has also been seen to be positive in nature. By eating frequent meals, the body is not allowed to go onto starvation mode and thereby the metabolism is maintained at a high since there it is made to experience a near constant availability of food and energy. Increased metabolism helps in burning the extra fat reserves in the body and hence helps in losing weight in a desirable manner. In summary, a high frequency smaller meal plan seems to be much more effective in reducing body fat percentage in comparison to the modern day three meal plan. This loss in fat percentage is ideal for weight loss as well as weight gain. Hence such a meal plan can be made an integral part of any weight management program.

Physical exercise as part of weight management plan

The second pillar in a healthy weight management program is regular physical exercise at the right intensity. It helps in increasing the energy output to create the deficit that is essential for weight loss to take place. In case weight gain is the goal, exercise provides stimulus forcing the body to grow to meet the additional demands placed on it. Whatever the goals may be, like a healthy weight management plan, a healthy exercise routine should include all the components – cardiovascular endurance, muscular endurance, muscular strength and flexibility.

1. Cardiovascular endurance exercises include all those exercises that involve repetitive movement of large muscle groups at a heart rate greater than resting heart rate. Exercises include running, jogging, swimming, cycling, rowing etc. The role of the cardiovascular system is to ensure efficient delivery of oxygen to different parts of the body. Performing regular cardio exercises not only improves the delivery mechanism of oxygen but also helps improve the efficiency of the vascular system and the exercising muscles to take up and utilize the oxygen delivered. Chronic adaptations as a result of cardio activities help in preventing cardiovascular and coronary artery diseases, metabolic disorders such as diabetes and metabolic syndrome and may also help in preventing certain forms of cancer.

2. Muscular endurance exercises help improve the endurance of different muscle groups in the body. Numerous activities of daily life involve repeated movements to be performed of a particular type and therefore utilize a particular muscle group. Improved muscular endurance helps in performing these movements without experiencing too much fatigue in the exercising muscle.

3. Muscular strength is the ability of a particular muscle to lift heavy loads. In daily life, the requirement to lift and carry heavy load often arises but infrequently. If the body is deconditioned to perform such a movement then there is risk of injury. Strength training exercises help in increasing lean muscle tissue in the body as well as improves the quality of

bone health by strengthening them. In such a manner it helps in performing activities of daily life.

4. Flexibility refers to pain free range of motion around a joint. This is one of the most neglected aspects of fitness and as age progresses it becomes the most important component. Flexibility training in the form of static stretches held for moderate to long durations helps in improving flexibility which then reduced the risk of injuries.

All these components of exercise are important in the context of weight management but more emphasis is directed towards exercises such as cardiovascular workouts. These exercises increase the heart rate in such a manner that the extra demands placed on the body force it to rely on stored energy reserves in the body. By careful planning of diet and intensity of workout it is possible to selectively utilize fat stored in the body for meeting the energy requirements. A balanced routine should include 40 minutes of moderate intensity aerobic activity for 3 to 4 times a week, strength training or resistance training of all the muscle groups at least twice a week and static stretching to improve flexibility should also be incorporated at least 2 to 3 times a week. Such a balanced workout leads to weight loss as well as improves overall physical fitness.

Rest & Relaxation

It is important to understand that the actual growth and development of the body does not take place while exercise is being performed. Exercise only provides the stimulus required for growth and development of tissues. The other ingredients that ensure that the purpose is fulfilled are balanced & nutritious diet and rest & relaxation. Post exercise when the body rests and is provided energy and nutrition is the time when the actual growth happens. At this stage the energy requirements should be met from within the fat stores for weight loss to take place. In case this is not done, the body will strip lean muscle tissue to meet the demands post by exercise. Also, in case enough rest is not provided to the body, the chance of overtraining leading to injury increases manifold. Adequate amount of rest and relaxation also helps in maintaining hormonal balance in the body. This is also crucial for healthy weight management.

Mental attitude

A perfectly designed diet plan or a perfectly designed exercise routine is of no use if the individual for whom it is designed is not able to adhere to it. This is where the role of a positive mental attitude comes into picture. Psychological factors play an important role in weight management than is generally imagined. In fact adherence to any plan is solely dependent on the attitude a person carries towards the lifestyle alteration that is being imposed as part of the plan. In case the weight management program is looked at as a set of limitations or restrictions that is forced, the chances of adherence in the short run as well as over a period of time diminish significantly. On the contrary an individual adopting a positive attitude looks at the program as a new positive lifestyle which is embraced with vigour and excitement.

Yoga for weight management

'Yoga' is derived from '*yuj*' in Sanskrit which means 'to unite'. Originating in ancient India, it is a unique combination of mental, physical as well as spiritual disciplines. This union that yoga refers to is the union of the individual with the universal. Yoga is believed to have originated more than 25,000 years ago and contrary to common knowledge it is not just a sequence of poses and postures for improving health and fitness. It is an ancient science that includes tools such as *pranayama* or breathing methods and techniques, meditation also called *dhyana* and finally physical postures or *asanas.*

The modern form of yoga is believed to have begun with Parliament of Religions convened in Chicago in the year 1893. In the convention *Swami Vivekanand* had a deep impact on the thinking of the audience. In subsequent tours in the United States he promoted various aspects of yoga. These talks and lectures led to yoga shedding the tag of a purely religious practice and being accepted by the western world. In the years since then health benefits emanating through regular yogic practices have been researched, documented and published all over the world. It is estimated that in the US alone more than 25 million people practice yoga on a regular basis.

The myriad benefits of yoga include physiological benefits such as improved flexibility, increased strength, better posture, weight loss, effective breathing, stronger immune system, improved bone strength and improvement in medical conditions such as migraine and insomnia; psychological benefits include stress relief, greater awareness, improved energy levels and an overall feeling of inner peace. Yoga is quite efficient in weight loss as well. It advocates a multi dimensional approach that incorporates physical, emotional and spiritual components and does not superficially work on eliminating the symptoms alone. The root cause of the problem is targeted through yoga to deal with the weight problem. It therefore involves detoxification, increasing metabolism, achieving hormonal balance, improving observation & awareness and cardiovascular endurance. Certain forms of yoga prescribe movements done at a rapid pace in a sequential manner that elevates heart rate to moderate or high levels and in such a manner mimic cardiovascular activities. This is very similar to circuit training which is a form of strength training where each muscle group is exercises one after the other without any rest. Such workout principles help in weight loss since heart rate is maintained at a moderate to high level for considerable duration. Apart from the *asanas* that are practiced, *kriyas* such as *kapalbhati* done at a vigorous intensity provides a good cardiovascular endurance workout. Different *asanas* also have different effects on the mind as well. Certain movements performed at a particular pace are known to provide calmness, while other movements help in boosting energy levels. Yoga *asanas* also improve thyroid and pituitary health and balanced secretion of hormones helps in improving metabolism to suit the body's requirements. Other benefits such as reduction in anxiety and detoxification of the body indirectly help in losing weight in a healthy manner. The psychological benefits such as improved awareness and sense of calmness help in immensely improving adherence to weight management program since they bring about a positive attitude towards the entire process.

Meditation for weight management

Meditation refers to the process of reflection and contemplation that helps in calming the mind and in this way relieves stress and anxiety. It has been commonly linked with religion and prayer across many cultures since ancient times. It is often thought of as a tool to improve concentration and as an aid to attaining peace of mind, a path to God and spirituality. Meditation is commonly done by mental exercises that include concentrated breathing, single point focussing as well as chanting. In some cultures it is performed by being completely detached from external worldly contacts while in others the person may interact with the outside world while practicing meditation.

Meditation has developed over centuries and across cultures and civilizations. There is no one form of meditation that fits all the requirements and is ideal for each and everyone practicing it. Which form suits whom depend on factors like state of mind, personality traits and external surroundings. The meditation form that should be practiced is the one in which the person feels most comfortable rather than going after something which is perceived by people in close contact to be most helpful. There is no one single source or authority or text that is referred to for meditation practices. Numerous different forms have evolved over ages each having certain distinct characteristics. A high proportion of these forms though, involve awareness of breath as the underlying platform on which meditation is practiced. Different types of meditation include the following:

1. *Mindfulness meditation* is a popular practice in the West in which awareness of the surroundings is not blocked out. The idea in this practice is to allow all the thoughts to flow into the mind without focusing on any single one of them. This form does not necessarily require quiet and peaceful surroundings and can be performed anywhere. Breathing like most meditation forms is important but is not the primary and sole element. It is a form which is suited to beginners who may find concentrating and blocking out thoughts to focus on nothingness extremely difficult.

2. *Focused meditation* involves focusing on a single thought throughout the practice session. The point of focus can be internal like an imagined object and can also be external in nature like a chant. The emphasis is not on the thought but

on the process of maintaining concentration and not losing focus.

3. *Spiritual meditation* is a form which is closely interlinked with religion and is suited to individuals who offer prayers as part of their daily rituals. The emphasis is on communication and interaction with God and union with the Universal.

4. *Trance based meditation* is an advanced form of spiritual meditation that involves reaching a state of trance by losing self control induced by usage of intoxicating substances. Since the person practicing this form of meditation may not have any memory of the experience, it has a very limited usage, if any, on daily life.

5. *Movement meditation* is a form in which the practice involves constant movement. These movements can be slow & rhythmic in nature such as swaying of the body. These gentle movements are believed to have a calming influence on the mind.

6. *Other forms of meditation* include mantra meditation, transcendental meditation, *kundalini* meditation, *Qi gong* meditation and *Zazen* meditation. Each of them originating in different ages and different parts of the world; differing in the way they are practiced and in terms of their end objectives as well.

Since it is not an exact science, the benefits of meditation cannot be directly and objectively measured. Interest in the scientific community has increased immensely as a result of observations, but studies and research has not determined conclusive proof of benefits derived from meditation. Physical benefits include elimination of stress leading to improvement in conditions such as hypertension and diabetes. The vibrations released are also known to have the added effect of diminishing the negative impact of the disease. Meditation is known to reduce the level of Cortisol and hence reduces stress levels; it also reduces the accumulation of lactic acid which is associated with anxiety. Meditation helps in breath control thereby reducing heart rate and helping the body fight against hypertension; it helps to improve immunity, provides balance to the hormonal system, improves fertility, reduces cholesterol level and helps in weight loss.

While weight loss cannot be directly achieved through meditation it has a more important role to play than any other parameter including physical exercise and diet & nutrition. Meditation does not burn fat in the body but it provides a frame of mind and attitude that is crucial for the efficient functioning of the tools that result in weight loss. Without a positive frame of mind adherence to the weight management program is practically impossible. Meditation helps in identifying the root cause of the weight problem and it does not superficially work on the symptoms of the problem. Even if an individual on a weight loss program is able to achieve weight loss, it may not be sustainable and permanent in case the root cause is not tackled. Meditation helps in improving self control and thereby increases determination that helps in adhering to the program. Moreover, the positive attitude with which the program is adopted magnifies the benefits that may be derived. From the psychological perspective of filling in voids, people have a tendency to go on binges – commonly termed as emotional eating. Meditation helps by working on elimination of desire itself helping the individual practicing it to remain unaffected by the pressures of daily home and work life. The positive attitude that is manifested helps to attain a balance in life. This balance prevents excessive emotions either positive or negative. The person thus practicing experiences an ever prevalent calmness irrespective of the external environment and the alterations that these parameters may undergo. While meditation objectively may not lead to weight loss in the conventional sense, it empowers the individual with a positive attitude – the most useful tool in attaining any weight loss goal.

Meditation also provides numerous psychological benefits. It helps ease stress & anxiety as mentioned earlier. A person becomes calm & composed and is able to visualize the external world with detachment helping in decision making process. Meditation also recharges and provides a feeling of rejuvenation which increases efficiency of all work that the person indulges in. Practicing meditation on a regular basis provides greater mental control that helps in curbing fluctuations in mood and emotion. The spiritual benefits that are derived from regular practice of meditation are manifested in the attitude of kindness and compassion towards others. Union of mind, body and soul leads to an infinite source of love. All these benefits from meditation practice helps produce a balanced personality unfazed by external events and conditions.

Conclusion

For a successful weight management program it is imperative that all these components or pillars be incorporated. When these pillars are not in sync the chances of success of these plans reduces considerably. In fact, neglecting any one of these components may compromise short term as well as long term health and wellness. On the other hand when the wavelengths of the efforts do not match it is very unlikely that the weight management goals are achieved. A positive attitude towards a weight management program that includes a well rounded physical fitness routine, a balanced diet & nutrition plan and sufficient rest & relaxation is almost a guarantee to achieving long term and sustainable weight loss.

Eat 6 Small Meals A Day

Benefits of eating six small meals a day versus 3 large meals

Understanding the human body

We are all aware that a weight management system plays an extremely crucial role in achieving health & fitness goals for each and every individual. Whether the goal is to lose weight or gain weight, to train for faster sprints or elite marathons, or whether it is to simply enjoy a healthy & positive lifestyle, diet and proper nutrition are cornerstones for a successful wellness plan.

Before we delve into what type of weight management plan is beneficial under what circumstances, let us first try and understand the human body and how it functions. Our body is made up of the following major components – bones, organs, fat, lean muscle tissue and water. Through a process called Body Composition Analysis we can determine the individual percentages of each of these components. Simple portable machines working on principles such as bioelectric impedance analysis and ultrasound are available which provide you the result within a few seconds. Each day newer technologies debut in the market providing more accurate results at cheaper costs. Even traditional methods such as skin-fold measurements using calipers are pretty accurate if performed properly. Understanding the body is the first step in the design of a health & fitness program, and these methods help us do this exact thing.

Out of these constituent components of the body only fat and lean muscle mass tissue are measured quantities that we aim to alter through a weight management program. If the goal is to lose weight, then we aim to reduce the amount of fat – both visceral (fat around the organs, typically the abdominal fat) & subcutaneous (under the skin, and distributed all over the body). Typically we refer to this process as healthy weight loss or fat loss. If the goal is to gain weight, then we aim to increase the amount of lean muscle mass while still maintaining or in some cases even slightly increasing the fat percentage in the body. For most people goals can be categorized into one of these two groups.

Any program that works upon changing other parameters in the body in all probability will compromise health of the individual participating in the program. For example, a weight loss gadget that gained widespread popularity was the sauna belt. As promised in all the marketing & advertising campaigns, it resulted in immediate weight loss. Within a short duration the person using the belt was able to lose weight as well as quite a few centimeters; and by short duration we mean minutes and not weeks! However, a closer inspection leads you to the crux of the functionality. It was working on dehydrating the body, essentially making you sweat and lose weight by losing water. This we can categorically state is not a healthy method to weight loss. No doubt, weight loss is achieved, but it is through dehydration and not through fat loss which is desired. Weight management plans are pretty much the most marketed products in the world each with the promise of rapid weight loss or weight gain as the case may be. However, calling a plan a product itself is the beginning of the problem. It is not something that is a one size fits all solution. Each individual is different and therefore a weight management plan has to be necessarily customized according to the specific needs of the individual.

The essential components of a weight management program aiming to achieve and maintain an optimum weight and level of health include: physical fitness, balanced & nutritious diet, adequate amount of rest and finally, mental relaxation & attitude. Each component is equally important and needs to be taken into consideration while designing a health & wellness program. In this particular section we shall be concentrating on weight management through proper nutrition.

What do you mean by a weight management diet plan?

The role of a good meal plan in achieving health goals cannot be over emphasized. It is one of the important pillars of a good health & wellness program. Unfortunately many people mistakenly consider it as the only pillar, convenience and control over parameter perhaps being the reasons.

A good nutritious and balanced diet goes a long way in ensuring long term good health. But what exactly do we mean by such a plan? To answer this question, we shall break up the problem into parts, starting with components of diet.

Components of diet

Our diet is composed of hundreds of different nutrients each of them having an important function or role to play in the sustenance of a healthy life. Simply put, a nutrient is a substance in our food that provides necessary nourishment. It may help in the growth of the body, provide energy for performance of daily functions, or promote optimal health and function. Some of these nutrients are deemed essential when the body by itself is not able to provide these nutrients or is not able to provide them in sufficient quantities. We generally classify the nutrients on the basis of their function. They can be broadly categorized into the following sections:

1. Energy nutrients
   a. Carbohydrates – principal source of energy
   b. Proteins – building blocks of life, essential for tissue growth and repair
   c. Fats – energy dense molecules storing energy in the body

2. Vitamins
   a. Vitamin A, C, D, K, E, Thiamine, Riboflavin etc. – each essential for one or more of numerous biochemical reactions in the human body

3. Minerals
   a. Calcium, Iron, Zinc, Sodium, Potassium etc. – catalysts for one or more of numerous biochemical reactions taking place in the body

4. Others
   a. Water – temperature regulator as well as nutrient & hormone transport mechanism

    b. Fiber – indigestible carbohydrates playing an impor-
tant role in digestion

Each of the aforementioned nutrients has multiple functions (only the most important functions have been mentioned here) and deficiency or even excess of these nutrients in the body may be harmful. It is therefore extremely important to follow a balanced diet as part of a weight management plan.

Balanced Diet

A pertinent question that arises at this stage is how we know how much of each nutrient is required by our body. The answer is given by standards such as RDA (Recommended Dietary Allowance), DRI (Dietary Reference Intakes), AI (Adequate Intake), EAR (Estimated Average Requirement) and DV (Daily Value). After extensive research across populations scientists across the world have developed these standards. They basically prescribe the quantities for intake of all these nutrients on a daily basis; variable parameters such as age and sex are taken into account. These standards themselves are not static and undergo changes on the basis of in depth research and analysis happening continuously.

A balanced weight management diet is one which provides all the nutrients in adequate quantities to maintain a balance at the same time works towards the weight goals of the program. It means that each of the specific nutrients should be consumed in quantities required to balance that which is used up by the body for the performance of daily functions as well as that which may be lost in the process. In general, non–energy nutrients such as vitamins and minerals should be consumed as per the standards prescribed. However, individuals may have variations in energy nutrients (carbohydrates, proteins & fats) depending upon their health and fitness goals. Even in these cases the meal plan should incorporate around 50 to 60% energy being provided through carbohydrates, 20 to 30% energy through fats and 15 to 20% through proteins. This ensures that while energy requirements of the body are met, simultaneously the energy nutrients are present in the correct quantities so that they are able to fulfill their other functions as well. In a nutshell the following points can be kept in mind for a balanced weight management meal plan:

1. All the micro nutrients – vitamins & minerals are consumed as per Daily Value range

2. Percentages of energy compounds – carbohydrate, protein and fat are as per suggested range

3. Adequate amount of water should be consumed – approximately 2 to 3 liters per day; this may increase depending upon environmental parameters such as temperature, humidity and altitude

4. Fiber is extremely important for digestion and adequate amounts should be consumed as part of the diet plan – roughly 25 to 35 grams per day

Key steps in the preparation of a diet plan

In this section we provide a step by step set of guidelines that should be used in the preparation of a weight management meal plan.

Step 1 – Understand the profile of the individual

The profile of an individual is the primary element required in the preparation of the plan. The plan for a 22 year old athlete will be very different from that of a 60 year old veteran. Similarly, it will be different for an adult woman in comparison to a man. Finally, health history and profile is extremely important to capture prior to preparation of the plan. Someone with a specific condition like rheumatoid arthritis or a deficiency such as that of Vitamin A will have a drastically different plan in comparison to someone who is not affected by these conditions.

Step 2 – Understand the health & fitness goals

The goal of an endurance athlete such as a long distance runner will be very different from that of a sprinter. In a similar vein, an obese individual looking to lose weight has a completely different fitness goal in comparison to a complete ectomorph trying to gain weight. Diet plan for these individuals will be very different owing to their varied fitness goals.

Step 3 – Understand the dietary preferences and lifestyle pattern

A perfect weight management meal plan is of no use in case the individual for whom it was prepared is not able to follow it. In case a vegan is prescribed a plan wherein protein requirements are met through meat products, it is highly improbable that the plan will be successful. Not only is the content of the plan important but also the extent to which it can be followed. A plan is doomed to fail in case it demands an individual to make certain lifestyle changes that may not be possible to incorporate. For example, a person working in an organization has late working hours and goes to sleep at 3:00 am. The diet plan prescribes a meal at say 5:00 am in the morning; it is unlikely that the person will change his current job and profile for the sake of such a rigid plan.

Step 4 – Calculate the caloric requirement

This is the step where the mathematical calculations begin. Despite whatever scientific studies get published every day, there is one basic rule that cannot be violated. It is a natural extension from the law of conservation of energy.

IF *Energy Input > Energy Output* THEN *result will be Weight Gain*

IF *Energy Input < Energy Output* THEN *result will be Weight Loss*

By energy output we mean the total energy that the body burns during the entire day. This is a summation of the following parameters:

1. Resting Metabolic Rate (RMR) – is the total energy that the body burns in a state of complete rest. This energy is required for essential body functions, like respiration.

2. Cost of activity (COA) – is the energy that the body burns due to daily routine activities. A software professional will be burning far fewer calories during work in comparison to a manager supervising an oil rig.

3. Cost of exercise (COE) – is the total energy expended in physical workouts and exercises. A 60 year old leading a sedentary lifestyle performing limited physical exercise such as walking for half an hour burns fewer calories in

comparison to a 25 year old running regularly for an hour each day.

4. Thermic effect of food (TEF) – is the energy required for digestion. A meal comprising of a high percentage of protein will require more energy to digest in comparison to a meal rich in fat or simple carbohydrates.

There are a few other parameters such as active and adaptive thermogenesis which have a relatively small contribution and are difficult to calculate. The net sum of these parameters is the total energy expended during the day and is the measure of Energy Output.

By energy input we mean the energy released in the body as a result of metabolism of food. The input depends on 2 parameters – firstly, what we eat and secondly, how much we eat. In the previous section we had discussed different energy nutrients. Each molecule of these nutrients provides exact number of calories:

1. 1 gram of Carbohydrate gives 4 calories

2. 1 gram of Protein gives 4 calories

3. 1 gram of Fat gives 9 calories

4. 1 gram of Alcohol gives 7 calories (generally kept out of consideration)

As can be expected, a gram of fat provides more than double the energy that is provided by a gram of protein or carbohydrate. Therefore, greater the percentage of energy nutrients within the meal greater will be the calorie content.

The difference between the energy input and energy output is called energy excess or deficit as the case may be. Now, to calculate the calorie requirement, we need to first understand that 1 pound of fat is roughly equivalent to 3,500 calories. Therefore, to gain or lose 1 pound of fat we need to achieve an excess or deficit of 3,500 calories. As is evident, this may be done over any length of time. For healthy weight gain or weight loss, it is suggested that the body should not undergo more than 2 pounds of change, thus ensuring that drastic and sudden changes are avoided. This is essential not only from a physical point of view but a hormonal point of view as well.

In case we want to lose 1 pound of fat on a weekly basis, then on a daily basis we need to create a deficit of approximately 500 calories. By doing our calculations, if we find that the daily energy output is 2,000 calories, then the diet within the weight management system should be made such that it provides 1,500 calories as input. By applying this process, we are able to arrive at the exact calorie requirement from the meal plan.

Step 5 – Finalize the frequency and timing of the meals

The timing of meals should be such that it takes into account the following parameters:

1. Time of getting up
2. Time of going to sleep
3. Time of workout/exercise
4. Other specific times that cannot be altered for weight management plan adherence

Barring a few manageable changes, not much should be expected to be altered in the lifestyle of the person for whom the plan is being made. At the initial stage at least, this method will increase the chances of adherence. Pre-workout and post-workout meals play an extremely crucial role in deciding what energy substrate is being utilized for meeting the increased energy demands. Moreover, they also determine whether stored energy is being utilized for the purpose or the immediate input is being utilized for providing the energy. The decision is directly derived from the goals of the program and therefore it is imperative that all the steps are followed in the preparation of the diet plan. The frequency of the meals in the weight management plan is discussed in detail in the next section.

Step 6 – Design a balanced diet meeting the above requirements

Once we have calculated the energy requirements and have arrived at the frequency and timings of the meals, the diet plan can be populated. Nutritional information regarding generic products such as whole grains and vegetables are readily available in published resources. For off the shelf products, all the information is clearly available in the nutrition data, providing which has been made mandatory. A certain amount of mixing and matching is required and at the end of this iterative process we arrive at a plan that meets all the requirements.

6 small meals versus a 3 meal plan

Once we have understood the basic concepts of a balanced diet within the structure of a weight management system, we can now analyze in detail the pros and cons of meal plans of varying frequency. In general, we can divide meal plans into two categories – high frequency small meal plan and low frequency large meal plan.

Since childhood during the formative years, we had been put in the habit of eating 3 meals on a daily basis – breakfast, lunch and dinner. On some days a snack may have been added here and there but this had been the pattern for numerous years. Breakfast usually meant consuming something small but energy rich, something readily available or something that could be prepared quickly. Lunch was always something that could be munched upon on the go, while dinner was the defining family meal, when everyone could sit down together after a hard day's work. Naturally this was the most enjoyable meal and perhaps the heaviest meal of the day. This matched not only our lifestyle but also that of other members of the family. The three square meals were ingrained as a concept in our dietary patterns.

However, the concept of high frequency small meals is catching up. There is no specific magic number but a 6 meal plan fits in well in our daily routine. That does not mean that a 5 meal or a 7 meal plan cannot be followed. The emphasis is on smaller meals taken more number of times during the day in a manner such that the gap between the traditional 3 meals – breakfast, lunch and dinner can be cut down.

Composition of 6 meal plan

Following all the steps as part of designing a healthy & balanced weight management meal plan, a generic 6 meal plan can be as following:

Meal 1 – Breakfast – As the name suggests it is the meal that literally 'breaks a fast'. It is the most important meal of the day and should comprise high energy foods to provide that energy punch required after a gap of almost 8 hours since the previous meal. A healthy mix of complex carbohydrates (those which release energy slowly over a period of time), healthy fat and proteins along with a vitamin & mineral boost through a fruit salad is ideal. Not only will such a meal be balanced in most regards, but will also provide the necessary energy required during the initial half of the day.

Meal 2 – Mid morning snack – It is essentially a snack the purpose of which is to reduce the gap between breakfast and lunch. This can simply be slices of carrot along with a nice low fat dip as accompaniment. The purpose is to cut out the gap and therefore the ensuing hunger pangs that may lead to overeating during lunch.

Meal 3 – Lunch – The afternoon meal should be well balanced comprising all essential macro nutrients as well as predominant set of micro nutrients. Ample nourishment along with appropriate energy through complex carbohydrates is the goal of this meal. Lean protein source such as grilled chicken, a decent serving of brown rice along with a bowl of vegetable salad dressed with olive oil is a good combination.

Meal 4 – Late afternoon/Evening snack – Like meal 2 it bridges the gap between lunch and dinner. Meal content is similar and can also consist of some dry fruits such as almonds along with low fat cheese or yogurt.

Meal 5 – Pre/Post workout snack – Timing of this meal is dependent on workout timings around which timings of other meals can be shuffled. Meal content is also dependent on health & fitness goals. It can include fruit/vegetable smoothies along with a protein shake. In a nutshell, in case goal is to lose fat simple carbohydrates can be cut out to a certain extent in a manner such that the body gets enough energy but at the same time gets this energy through energy substrates stored in the body such as fat and glycogen. On the other hand, if increase in lean muscle tissue is the goal, it is important to provide an insulin spike during the anabolic window immediately post workout. Therefore, a combination of simple sugars to create the insulin spike and fast acting proteins such as whey should do the trick.

Meal 6 – Dinner – On similar lines as lunch, it should be well balanced providing nourishment. However, the carbohydrate intake can be restricted since, metabolism as well as energy requirements are at a decline. It is important to also ensure that there is a small gap before pushing off to sleep. Lean protein like grilled fish, a baked vegetable preparation with sauce is a decent option.

It is important to note that there is no magic number as discussed earlier. If possible, a couple of meals such as a small pre–dinner snack to avoid hunger pangs can be incorporated within the existing structure. However, enough care should be taken so that the suggested calorie requirement is not violated at any cost. An important disclaimer here is that this is a very general plan and may not necessarily apply to specific conditions and requirements. As has been mentioned earlier a good weight management meal plan is one which is customized and tailor made suited to the goals of the individual.

Benefits of 6 meal plan over a 3 meal plan

There are numerous benefits that are derived from breaking down 3 heavy meals into 6 lighter meals.

1. *Energy requirement matching* – The body does not require energy according to when we eat; rather we should eat to match the varying rate at which the body demands energy. Unless demanding activities like exercise routine is performed the body does not need energy in discrete shots. By breaking the heavy meals into smaller portions we provide energy to the body in a continuous manner, slowly and gradually. As can be expected, the excess carbohydrate gets converted to fat and gets stored in the body. Therefore, smaller meals are better at matching this energy requirement.

2. *Prevention of insulin spikes* – Whenever there is an increase in the level of circulating glucose in the blood stream as a

result of a heavy meal, the pancreas releases insulin which then promotes the movement of this glucose into the cells, both muscle and fat cells. All cells in take up glucose from the blood to meet varied energy demands. Immediately after a meal though the fat, liver and muscle cells take up more than they require so that insulin levels can drop back to normal levels. When a heavy meal is consumed insulin spike stays on for longer resulting in storage of carbohydrates. Initially this is stored in the form of glycogen (a long chain glucose molecule) but due to limited storage capacity, excess amount starts getting converted into fat. To prevent this conversion from happening lighter meals are preferred; since calorie requirements are still to be met, greater will be the desired number of meals during the day.

3. *Promotion of utilization of stored energy reserves* – The body stores energy in the form of glucose in the blood, glycogen in the liver & muscles and finally fat in the fat cells. Whenever, energy is required it is met from either of these sources. Insulin as described above helps and promotes the cells to utilize the carbohydrate received from the meal. Whenever extra carbohydrates enter the body through a heavy meal, the body stops depending on fat reserves stored in the body for energy production. Moreover, the extra carbohydrate again gets converted into fat. Not only is the body storing extra fat, it is also depending lesser and lesser on already stored fat in the body. This is another important factor that highlights the importance of the 6 meal plan.

4. *Prevention of sluggishness post heavy meals* – A common experience after a heavy meal is the ensuing sluggishness. The main reason for this is that to digest the large quantities of food the body is made to work that much harder. By switching to smaller meals these peaks and troughs are avoided.

5. *Decreases craving and unplanned eating* – By cutting out the large time gaps between the meals cravings that arise due to calorie controlled meals are prevented. Moreover, unplanned eating is avoided since eating a healthy snack is any

which ways a part of the diet plan. Thus, by design themselves, 6 meal plans increase the chances of complete adherence to the weight management program.

6. *Prevents overeating during main meals* – In continuation with the previous benefit, uncontrolled hunger pangs that may lead to overeating during main meals are avoided. By having a small salad or vegetable smoothie prior to main meal we can prevent uncontrolled eating that may happen in case there is a long gap after the previous meal. We are then in a position to enjoy healthier options as planned.

7. *Increased metabolism* – It is commonly believed that more frequent meals help increase the metabolism rate. Whenever, meals are skipped or there is a huge time gap between meals, the body tends to go into a kind of starvation mode, thereby reducing the rate at which it uses up stored energy reserves of the body. Frequent meals specifically those rich in proteins require energy for digestion. This is where thermic effect of food also comes into play, which is the work being done by the body during this entire process. Increased metabolism will help burn the extra fat reserves stored in the body. An important disclaimer here is that this phenomenon of increased metabolism is something that does not have a very concrete scientific base. The theory is based on the empirical studies conducted on a limited sample size. On the contrary, some researchers believe that the only way in which the metabolic rate of the body can be altered is through an increase or decrease in lean muscle tissue. Through regular exercise specifically resistance training, lean muscle tissue increases which requires energy to maintain. An increase of 1 pound of lean muscle tissue can increase the metabolic rate by up to 60 calories. Thus exercising regularly is a sure shot method to increase metabolism, and therefore should supplement the diet within a weight management program.

8. *Lower levels of LDL cholesterol* – Like in the case of metabolism, only empirical studies have shown lowering effects of 6 meal plans on LDL cholesterol, considered the bad

cholesterol. The study was conducted on two sample groups, one on a 6 meal plan and the other group on a 3 meal plan. At the end of it, the 6 meal group showed significantly lower LDL cholesterol levels.

Summarizing the aforementioned points, small but frequent meals such as that proposed by 6 meal plans, help in reducing body fat percentages. Whether the goal is to gain weight or to reduce weight, a reduction of stored fat in the body is desired in most cases. This is precisely what these meal plans help in achieving.

Caveats of 6 meal plans that need to be addressed

Despite all the benefits provided by 6 meal plans, it is important to take care of a few important points while implementing such a diet plan.

1. *Meeting calorie goals* – Whether it is a 6 meal plan or a 3 meal plan, energy excess will lead to weight gain and an energy deficit will lead to weight loss. This is the inviolable rule that overrides everything. For an individual aiming to lose weight, not only is consuming more calories than planned counterproductive to the program, consuming much lesser calories than planned can not only result in increasing body fat, it may also be harmful in the long run. There is a possibility that during fasting this may occur with people with high fat percentages and lower activity levels.

2. *Lack of dietary control* – Some people find it extremely difficult to stop eating once they start to. For such people, a 6 meal plan may not be ideal, since they have a tendency to overeat during each of the meals. Consequently, at the end of the day, the number of calories consumed will be far greater than planned. This will lead to an energy excess and therefore weight gain. The entire purpose of the meal plan thus gets thwarted. Psychological experts propose that people who face such problems should take small but disciplined steps initially and then over a period of time embark on stricter and more rigorous plans.

3. *Customize implementation of plan* – It may not be feasible for everyone to follow such a plan to the word. It is better to take a few steps in the right direction than not move at all. For example, it may not be possible for a working professional to prepare and carry separate meals as per the 6 meal plan. In such a situation, even a meal split into two parts plays a good enough part. Improvise and customize the program but adhere to it once it has been planned.

4. *Ensure balanced diet* – At times it may happen that to ensure smaller quantity meals as part of the 6 meal plan, adequate attention may not be paid to ensure a balanced diet. Some important nutrient may get left out on a perennial basis as a result of this. Deficiency may consequently arise, which is absolutely undesirable.

On the whole, the benefits derived from small but high frequency meal plan are significant. It is not something that is only restricted to specific fitness & health goals. As a generic meal program structure it is highly advisable. The key is to ensure that it is followed in entirety and not in components. As is always the case, adherence to the plan defines the results that may be achieved through it. Inherently '6 meal plans' have a structure that promotes active adherence and make it easier for an individual to follow, thereby leading to long term health & wellness.

Body goals diary

_____

_____

_____

_____

_____

_____

_____

_____

_____

_____

_____

_____

_____

_____

Body goals diary

_____

_____

_____

_____

_____

_____

_____

_____

_____

_____

_____

_____

_____

_____

_____

Body goals diary

_____

_____

_____

_____

_____

_____

_____

_____

_____

_____

_____

_____

_____

_____

_____

_____

Body goals diary

_____

_____

_____

_____

_____

_____

_____

_____

_____

_____

_____

_____

_____

_____

_____

Body goals diary

_____

_____

_____

_____

_____

_____

_____

_____

_____

_____

_____

_____

_____

_____

_____

Body goals diary

_____

_____

_____

_____

_____

_____

_____

_____

_____

_____

_____

_____

_____

_____

Body goals diary

Body goals diary

_____

_____

_____

_____

_____

_____

_____

_____

_____

_____

_____

_____

_____

_____

Body goals diary

_____

_____

_____

_____

_____

_____

_____

_____

_____

_____

_____

_____

_____

_____

Body goals diary

_____

_____

_____

_____

_____

_____

_____

_____

_____

_____

_____

_____

_____

_____

Body goals diary

_____

_____

_____

_____

_____

_____

_____

_____

_____

_____

_____

_____

_____

_____

_____

Body goals diary

_____

_____

_____

_____

_____

_____

_____

_____

_____

_____

_____

_____

_____

_____

Body goals diary

_____

_____

_____

_____

_____

_____

_____

_____

_____

_____

_____

_____

_____

_____

Body goals diary

_____

_____

_____

_____

_____

_____

_____

_____

_____

_____

_____

_____

_____

_____

_____

Body goals diary

_____

_____

_____

_____

_____

_____

_____

_____

_____

_____

_____

_____

_____

_____

_____

Body goals diary

_____

_____

_____

_____

_____

_____

_____

_____

_____

_____

_____

_____

_____

_____

Body goals diary

_____

_____

_____

_____

_____

_____

_____

_____

_____

_____

_____

_____

_____

_____

Body goals diary

_____

_____

_____

_____

_____

_____

_____

_____

_____

_____

_____

_____

_____

_____

Body goals diary

_____

_____

_____

_____

_____

_____

_____

_____

_____

_____

_____

_____

_____

_____

_____

Body goals diary

_____

_____

_____

_____

_____

_____

_____

_____

_____

_____

_____

_____

_____

About the author

C. T. Pam is not a physician, rather she is a regular person who has explored many avenues of eating healthy and finding a healthy lifestyle balance. After a car accident in 2010 left her unable to continue running, she found a work-life balance that has helped her maintain a healthy lifestyle. C. T. Pam has a B.A. in Political Science and Studio Art, an MBA with a entrepreneurship concentration and is currently pursuing a doctoral degree with a research focus in Entrepreneurship.

Book description

This book includes sound advice and facts regarding

- Introduction to weight management
- Choosing meal portions

While this book doesn't intend to tell the reader the best way to lead a healthy lifestyle, the author advises the reader to take away items that he or she can realistically achieve. You won't lose 50 pounds overnight, and you will have an opportunity to explore options that might benefit your physical, emotional and lifestyle needs. This book includes pages for the reader to record their goals and progress.

Volume 3 is an excerpt from Adopting a healthy lifestyle (1-884711-34-0)

Also available from Innovative Publishers

Introduction to the Paleo diet. (978-1884711466)

Introduction to the Paleo diet + 200 recipes (1884711820)

Love is… (978-1884711138)

Extreme Betrayal (978-1884711084)

Beware the Bumble Bee (978-1884711091)

Doing business with the U. S. government (978-1884711107)

Visit http://innovative-publishers.com for ordering information

Find us online @

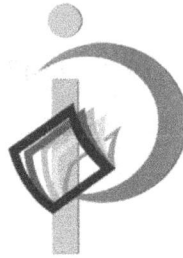

Innovative Publishers

 InnovaPub

 www.innovative-publishers.com

 pub@innovative-publishers.com

 http://innovativepublishers.blogspot.com/

 http://www.facebook.com/InnovativePublishers

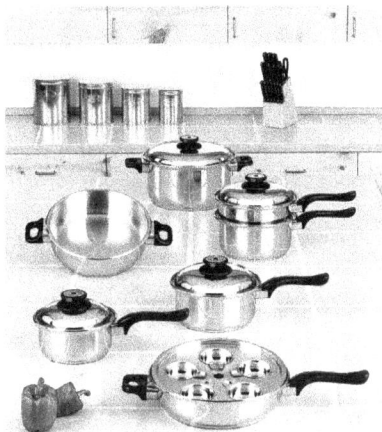

World's Finest™ 7-Ply Steam Control™ 17pc T304 Stainless Steel Cookware Set

Each piece is constructed of extra-heavy stainless steel and guaranteed to last a lifetime. Steam control valves make "waterless" cooking easy and the 7-ply construction spreads heat quickly and evenly, allowing one stack to cook. Cookware is also equipped with superbly styled phenolic handles resistant to heat, cold and detergents. Comes with a limited lifetime warranty. White box.

Suggested Retail Price : $2195.00

Item Number : GGKT17ULTRA

Set Contents

- 1.7Qt Covered Saucepan
- 2.5Qt Covered Saucepan
- 3.2Qt Covered Saucepan
- 7.5Qt Covered Roaster
- 11-3/8" Skillet, Double Boiler Unit With Capsule Bottom That You Can Also Use As An Extra 3Qt Saucepan
- 5 Egg Cups
- 5 Hole Utility Rack And High Dome Cover With Capsule Bottom So You Can Use As A Frypan
- Cover Fits Skillet Or Roaster

Features

- Extra-Heavy Stainless Steel Construction
- Heat-Resistant Phenolic Handles
- 7-Ply Construction

Limited Lifetime Warranty

» Estimated Case Weight : 36.55 Lbs.

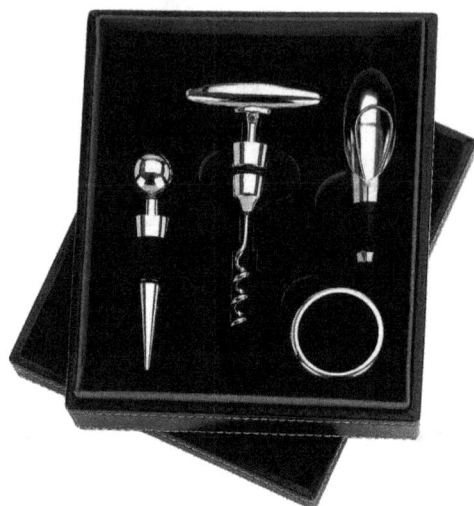

Wyndham House™ 4pc Wine Set in Storage Case

Wyndham House™ wine sets are a great compliment to any home bar, and are sure to add to the ease and elegance of wine presentations. Includes stainless steel wine spout, stainless steel wine ring, zinc alloy screw opener, and zinc alloy wine stopper. All enclosed in a 6-3/8" x 5-5/8" x 2-1/4" faux leather case.

Suggested Retail Price : $32.95

Next Ship Date : 01/05/2013

Item Number : GGKTWINE4

Features

- Stainless Steel Wine Spout
- Stainless Steel Wine Ring
- Zinc Alloy Screw Opener
- Zinc Alloy Wine Stopper
- 6-3/8" X 5-5/8" X 2-1/4" Faux Leather Case

Shipping Details

» Estimated Piece Weight : 1.10 Lbs.

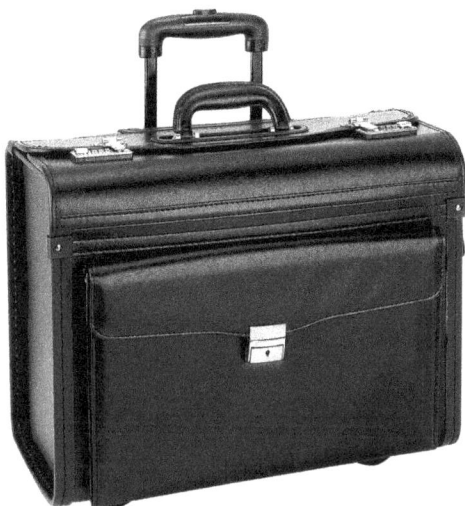

Embassy™ Sample/Pilot Case with Aluminum Trolley

Features PVC matte black exterior, rolling wheels, gunmetal combination locks, carrying handle, 2 exterior pockets, interior dividers, interior pockets, and pen holders. Measures 19" x 14" x 9".

Suggested Retail Price : $233.95

Number : BCPILOT3

Features

- Pvc Matte Black Exterior
- Rolling Wheels
- Gunmetal Combination Locks
- Carrying Handle
- 2 Exterior Side Pockets
- Interior Dividers & Pockets
- Pen Holders
- Measures 18" X 13" X 8"

Shipping Details

» Estimated Piece Weight : 8.70 Lbs.

To order products, go to the Innovative Publishers website and click Client specials. Clients receive up to 70% off the suggested retail price.

www.ingramcontent.com/pod-product-compliance
Lightning Source LLC
Chambersburg PA
CBHW060633280326
41933CB00012B/2030